STRENGTH TRAINING FOR TEEN BOYS

A Teen's Guide to Strength Training, Nutritional Mastery, and Mental Resilience for a Powerful, Confident, and Healthy Future

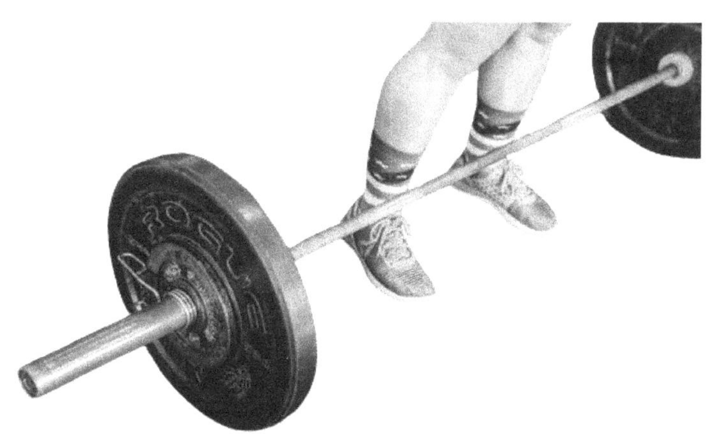

By Desmond T. Hall

Copyright © 2023 by Desmond T. Hall

All rights reserved. No part of this publication may be reproduced, stored in a retrieval system, or transmitted in any form or by any means, electronic, mechanical, photocopying, recording, or otherwise, without the prior written permission of the copyright owner, except for brief quotations in critical reviews and certain other noncommercial uses permitted by copyright law.

Declaimer ▲

This book is a work of nonfiction. Names, characters, places, and incidents are either the product of the author's imagination or are used fictitiously. Any resemblance to actual persons, living or dead, business establishments, events, or locales is entirely coincidental.

TABLE OF CONTENTS

INTRODUCTIONS 5

CHAPTER 1 6

Understanding the Basics 6

Why Strength Training is Important for Teens 7

Setting Realistic Goals.. 8

CHAPTER 2 11

Building a Strong Foundation....................................... 11

Fundamentals of Proper Nutrition 12

The Importance of Sleep for Recovery......................... 13

Body Awareness and Posture 13

CHAPTER 3 15

Getting Started with Exercises 15

Introduction to Bodyweight Exercises 16

Some Common Mistakes to Avoid When Doing
Bodyweight Exercises 18

Basic Resistance Training Techniques 19

Examples of Resistance Training Exercises for Teen Boys
.... 20

Proper Warm-up and Cool-down Routines 28

CHAPTER 4 30

Safety First: Guidelines and Precautions..................... 30

Understanding Your Body's Limits 31

Common Injuries and Prevention Strategies 32

Importance of Supervision and Form 33

CHAPTER 5 35

Strength Training for Sports and Fitness 35

Tailoring Workouts for Specific Sports 36

Cross-Training Benefits 37

Balancing Strength and Cardiovascular Fitness 38

CHAPTER 6 40

Mind and Body Connection 40

Mental Resilience and Confidence 41

Stress Management through Exercise 42

The Role of Strength Training in Mental Well-being .. 43

CHAPTER 7 44

Lifestyle Integration and Future Growth 44

Creating Sustainable Habits 45

Tracking and Celebrating Progress 46

Resources for Continued Learning and Growth 46

Tips for Staying Motivated To Continue Strength Training 47

CONCLUSION 49

Progress Tracker Journal 50

INTRODUCTIONS

Introducing "Strength Training for Teen Boys," an extensive guide created to assist male teenagers in realizing their maximum potential with the use of strength training. This book is about more than simply weightlifting; it's about fostering healthy habits, boosting self-esteem, and laying the groundwork for an active and healthy lifestyle.

Within, you'll discover:

- ✓ **Professional guidance**: Gain knowledge from seasoned experts who comprehend the special requirements and difficulties faced by teenage guys.
- ✓ **Easy-to-follow routines** that can be performed at home or the gym with little to no equipment—just your body weight—will help you achieve simple and effective fitness.
- ✓ **Put an emphasis on technique and safety**: Make sure your adolescent is safe by teaching them the right form and technique to minimize risks of injury and optimize outcomes.
- ✓ **Increased self-esteem**: As your teen begins to perceive and experience the advantages of strength training, assist them in developing self-confidence.
- ✓ **Lifelong fitness habits**: Help your adolescent cultivate a passion for physical activity and a long-term commitment to a healthy lifestyle.

Don't pass up the chance to bestow power and confidence on your adolescent kid. Get a copy of **"Strength Training for Teen Boys" right away**, and you may see him reach his greatest potential.

CHAPTER 1

Understanding the Basics

Strength training for teen males is a safe and effective technique to improve overall fitness, create stronger muscles, increase bone strength, improve mental health, minimize injury risk, and improve sports performance. To get these advantages, a strength training program must include the following components:

1. **Exercise Frequency and Duration**: Teens should engage in strength exercises for at least 20-30 minutes every day for the greatest effects. 2 or 3 days each week, with at least one day off in between. Working the primary muscular groups of the arms, legs, and core is essential.

2. **Exercise Methods**: Strength training may be done using free weights, weight machines, resistance bands, and bodyweight movements including push-ups, sit-ups, planks, and squats.

3. **Safety and Technique**: To maintain the safety and efficacy of strength training, proper supervision and coaching are required. Teens should concentrate on learning and practicing proper technique before progressively increasing the weight of their exercises.

4. **Advantages and Considerations**: Strength training improves not just physical health but also mental health, self-esteem, and athletic performance. It is critical to comprehend the possible benefits and drawbacks of strength training for adolescent guys.

Teen boys may safely and efficiently include strength training into their fitness regimen by following these instructions and knowing the fundamental concepts of strength training. This will result in increased overall health and well-being.

Why Strength Training is Important for Teens

Strength training is essential for teenagers because it provides several benefits that help to their general health and well-being. It helps them enhance their fitness, gain lean body mass, burn more calories, and strengthen their bones. Strength exercise can also improve mental health, raise self-esteem, and lower the chance of injury.

It also improves sports performance by improving strength, power, and speed, offering them a competitive advantage in their sporting endeavors.

Strength training has also been found to increase strength, balance, lipid profiles, fat-free mass, and personal self-esteem in children and adolescents, adding to their overall well-being.

Strength training, when done correctly and under supervision, may help youth grow muscular strength, enhance bone density, strengthen ligaments and tendons, and improve athletic performance. It also aids in the promotion of good blood pressure and cholesterol levels, the maintenance of a healthy weight, and the prevention of accidents.

Strength training in a teenager's routine not only improves their physical health but also instills lasting fitness habits, fosters the development of a love of exercise, and supports the maintenance of a healthy lifestyle for years to come.

Strength training allows kids to build important skills such as optimal movement patterns, address main muscle groups, and enhance muscular coordination, all of which are good to both physical and psychological development.

Setting Realistic Goals

Setting realistic goals for teen males' strength training is critical for their safety, success, and motivation. When setting objectives, it is critical to consider the following factors:

1. Frequency and Duration of Exercise: Teens should engage in strength exercises for at least 20-30 minutes each day. 2 or 3 days each week, with at least one day off in between. It is critical to work the primary muscular groups of the arms, legs, and core.

2. Exercise Methods: Strength training may be done with free weights, weight machines, resistance bands, and bodyweight movements including push-ups, sit-ups, planks, and squats.

3. Weight and repetitions: Teens should be able to perform three sets of 10 to 15 repetitions at each weight. This guarantees that they are employing a weight that they are capable of handling. If they can only complete three or five reps, the weight is too heavy and they will injure themselves.

4. Safety and Technique: To maintain the safety and efficacy of strength training, proper supervision and coaching are required. Teens should concentrate on learning and

practicing proper technique before progressively increasing the weight of their exercises.

5. Aesthetic Goals: It is critical for teenagers not to become obsessed with appearance. Strength training provides a cascade of physical and mental benefits, and it's critical to pay attention to nonaesthetic indicators such as new abilities learned and how they feel.

6. Long-Term Growth: Strength training should be seen as a journey rather than a race. It is critical to be patient with the body and mind, realizing that each individual is restricted by elements such as heredity and biology.

Teen males may safely and efficiently include strength training into their exercise regimen by setting realistic objectives that take these aspects into account, leading to increased overall health and well-being.

Some of the most typical mistakes teen guys make when setting strength training goals are as follows:

- Setting unrealistic or ambiguous objectives can lead to dissatisfaction and a lack of progress. Setting concise, attainable, and quantifiable objectives is essential for staying motivated and tracking progress.
- Inconsistency in Training, diet, and recuperation: Failure to maintain consistent in training, diet, and recuperation can stymie growth. Adherence to a well-structured training program is critical for reaching strength training goals.
- Ignoring Safety and Technique: Lifting larger weights without first focusing on good form and technique might increase the risk of injury. It is critical for long-term

success and safety to emphasize correct form and progressively increase weights.

- Inadequate Form: Choosing to lift bigger weights over maintaining proper form can lead to injuries and stymie growth. To guarantee successful and safe strength training, it is critical to focus on good form and technique.
- Too Much Weight: Underestimating the amount of weight you lift might result in poor technique and injury. Starting with modest weights and progressively progressing to greater loads as strength and technique develop is critical.
- Lack of Training Structure: Failure to adhere to a well-structured training program might stymie growth. It is critical to have a clear strategy and framework for training sessions in order to achieve strength training goals.

Teen males may create more effective and realistic strength training objectives by being aware of these typical blunders, resulting in safer and more successful training outcomes.

"Lift the weights, lift your spirit." Each rep brings you closer to being a stronger, unstoppable self. Keep going, champion!"

CHAPTER 2

Building a Strong Foundation

A solid foundation in teen strength training is critical for their safety, growth, and long-term development. It entails teaching basic motions, stressing safety and skill, and encouraging age-appropriate program design. To do this, it is critical to examine the following fundamental elements:

✓ **Fundamental Movements:** Basic actions such as lower body pushes, lower body pulls, upper body pushes, and upper body pulls help juvenile athletes build a firm foundation. Before teaching more complicated exercises, these motions should be learned to ensure competency and safety.

✓ **Exercise approaches:** To efficiently improve strength, use a variety of approaches such as bodyweight workouts, resistance bands, and light dumbbells. These approaches are appropriate for teenagers and aid in the establishment of a solid foundation for more advanced training.

✓ **Safety and Supervision**: Adequate supervision and education are essential for ensuring the safety and efficiency of teen strength training. To minimize accidents and enhance long-term success, coaches and trainers should focus safety, technique, and age-specific education

✓ **Program Design**: Building a firm foundation in teen strength training requires a well-structured training program that focuses on fundamental motions, safety, and age-appropriate workouts. This involves a focus on safety, technique, and age-appropriate training to avoid injuries and enhance long-term success.

By embracing these factors, teen males may lay a solid foundation in strength training, laying the groundwork for long-term development and improvement that is safe, effective, and successful.

Fundamentals of Proper Nutrition

Teen guys who engage in strength training require proper diet. It is critical to eat a well-balanced diet that contains all of the nutrients required for growth, development, and recuperation. Here are some nutritional fundamentals:

Consume a range of foods: Eating a variety of meals guarantees optimal nutritional intake. Fruits, vegetables, whole grains, lean protein, and healthy fats should all be included in a well-balanced diet.

Consume entire foods: entire foods are high in nutrients and contain important vitamins, minerals, and fiber. Fresh and frozen fruits and vegetables, entire grains, lean protein sources, and healthy fats are all examples.

Limit your intake of processed foods, which are generally heavy in calories, harmful fats, and added sugars. Limiting their consumption can help you maintain a healthy weight and lower your risk of chronic illnesses.

Maintain adequate hydration, digestion, and general health by drinking plenty of water. Aim for at least 8-10 glasses of water every day for adolescent guys.

Consume enough calories: Eating enough calories is essential for energy, development, and recuperation.

Strength training in adolescent males may demand more calories than their inactive counterparts.

The Importance of Sleep for Recovery

Sleep is essential for healing, especially after physical effort such as strength training. Several studies have shown that sleep is essential for healthy cognitive, motor, and physiological activities. Human growth hormone (HGH), which operates on many tissues to promote repair, recuperation, and development, is released by the body during sleep. Furthermore, sleep allows for the clearance of superfluous metabolic waste from brain cells, increases blood flow to cells, and transports vital oxygen and glycogen required for recuperation.

As it helps to muscle regeneration and general physical performance, good, quality sleep is one of the most effective ways to recuperate and recharge after training and exercise.

Furthermore, sleep aids memory formation and adds to future performance, making it necessary for cognitive processing and decision-making, both of which are critical for athletes.

Body Awareness and Posture

Body awareness and posture are critical components of teen guys' strength training. Developing strong body awareness and posture can help decrease injury risk, increase movement efficiency, and boost overall performance. Consider the following crucial points:

Body Consciousness: Body awareness is the ability to notice and comprehend one's own body's location, movement, and sensations. Body awareness may help youth understand how their bodies move and feel, resulting in higher movement quality and a lower chance of injury.

Posture and Movement: Good posture is critical for reducing stress on tissues, muscles, and joints and allowing the body to operate optimally. Good posture also encourages efficient movement, which lowers the chance of injury and improves overall performance.

Neuromuscular Connection: Body awareness is intimately linked to the neurological system, which governs movement. Body awareness helps the neurological system adapt and maintain new movement patterns, resulting in better posture and less muscular stress.

Body Awareness and Posture Exercises: Several exercises can assist build and enhance body awareness and posture. These exercises emphasize how you move rather than how much, how fast, or how hard to move.

Ergonomics and everyday chores: Improving body awareness may be accomplished via basic everyday chores such as altering one's sitting or standing posture. These minor adjustments can assist to increase kinesthetic awareness and produce a more robust body that is less prone to pain and dysfunction.

Postural Training is a type of exercise that focuses on improving posture and body awareness. It includes workouts that target major postural muscles including the core, back, and neck. Postural training can aid in the improvement of posture, the reduction of muscular stress, and the enhancement of overall performance.

CHAPTER 3

Getting Started with Exercises

To begin exercising, it's critical to first establish your fitness objectives, present physical condition, and any potential health concerns. When starting an exercise regimen, keep the following points in mind:

- **Determine Your Fitness Objectives and Health Status:** It is critical to analyze your fitness objectives and general health before beginning any workout program. Decide if you want to enhance your cardiovascular fitness, strength, flexibility, or a mix of the three. Consider any current health concerns or physical restrictions that may limit the kind of workouts you can do.
- **Consult a Doctor:** If you have any health issues or are new to exercise, it is best to seek the advice of a healthcare expert, such as a physician or a qualified fitness trainer. They can advise you on the best workouts to do based on your current health and fitness objectives.
- **Select the Correct Exercises**: Choose the best activities for your fitness goals and health evaluation. Cardiovascular activities (e.g., walking, cycling, or swimming) for improving heart health, strength training (e.g., weightlifting or bodyweight exercises) for muscle growth, and flexibility exercises (e.g., yoga or stretching routines) for boosting range of motion are examples of these.

- **Begin gradually and slowly. Increase Intensity:** When starting an exercise regimen, it's critical to start slowly and progressively increase the difficulty. This method helps to avoid injury while also allowing your body to adapt to the demands of exercise.
- **Emphasis on Form and Technique:** Prioritize appropriate form and technique whether doing weight training, cardiovascular activities, or flexibility programs. This guarantees that you get the most out of each workout while reducing your chance of damage.
- Rest and recuperation are essential components of every training routine. Allow time for your body to recuperate between exercises, and make sure you're receiving enough sleep to sustain your physical activity.
- **Continue to Be Consistent:** Exercise benefits require consistency. Aim to develop a consistent workout regimen that fits your schedule and lifestyle. This will help you gain momentum and form a habit of exercising.
- **Keep an eye on your progress:** Keep track of your progress by writing down your exercises, noting any gains in strength, endurance, or flexibility, and altering your exercise program as required to keep yourself challenged.

Introduction to Bodyweight Exercises

Bodyweight exercises are a sort of strength training in which the individual's own weight is used to produce resistance against gravity. Strength, power, endurance, speed, flexibility, coordination, and balance may all be improved with these workouts.

Bodyweight training has grown in popularity among both recreational and professional athletes due to the numerous benefits it provides, including greater fitness, reduced injury risk, and enhanced confidence.

Bodyweight exercises may be done anywhere, at any time, and do not require any equipment or a gym membership. They are an excellent choice for beginners since they give a strong basis for more advanced exercises and are easily adaptable to different fitness levels.

Bodyweight exercises can also be combined with other types of exercise, such as aerobic training or weightlifting, to create a well-rounded fitness regimen.

The advantages of bodyweight activities go beyond physical health. They can also aid in the development of mental toughness, willpower, and overall well-being. Bodyweight exercises need concentration, dedication, and perseverance, all of which may be applied to other aspects of life.

To begin with bodyweight exercises, evaluate your fitness objectives and health state, select the appropriate types of exercises, begin slowly and gradually build intensity, focus on good form and technique, integrate rest and recovery, stay consistent, and track your progress.

Bodyweight exercises can be performed in six different movement patterns:

- Bending
- Squatting
- Lunging
- Pushing
- Pulling
- Burpees

Some Common Mistakes to Avoid When Doing Bodyweight Exercises

There are numerous typical errors that people make while doing bodyweight exercises that they should avoid in order to get the most out of their workouts and limit their chance of injury. Here are some of the most typical mistakes to avoid:

- **Skipping the Warm-Up**: Starting an exercise without first warming up is a typical error that can result in injury or muscle cramping. Warming up for 5-10 minutes before every workout is vital to get the blood circulating into the muscles, ligaments, and joints.

- **Poor Range of Motion**: Another common error that can restrict the efficacy of bodyweight workouts is using a poor range of motion. To reap the maximum advantages of each exercise, it is critical to employ the proper range of motion. Push-ups, for example, should be performed low to the ground, whereas squats should be performed with your thighs parallel to the ground.

- **Neglecting good Form and Technique**: Prioritizing the amount of reps or sets above good form and technique can lead to injury and decreased effectiveness. To promote successful and safe bodyweight exercise, good form and technique must be prioritized.

- **Skipping the Cool-Down:** Another common error that can impede healing and cause discomfort is skipping the cool-down. A cool-down is essential to kick-start healing, relax muscles, prevent discomfort, and prepare to workout again as soon as possible.

- **Not advancing Over Time**: A frequent error that can restrict the efficacy of bodyweight workouts is not advancing over time. It is critical to gradually raise the difficulty of workouts in order to continue pushing the body and achieving development.

You may guarantee to get the most out of your bodyweight workouts by avoiding these frequent blunders, leading to enhanced fitness, reduced injury risk, and increased confidence. To promote successful and safe bodyweight training, it is critical to stress good form and technique, improve over time, and implement warm-up and cool-down exercises.

Bodyweight, free weights, resistance bands, or weight machines can all be used to execute basic resistance training techniques. These approaches aid in the development of physical strength and endurance. Some of the fundamental resistance training techniques are as follows:

1. **Bodyweight exercises**, such as push-ups, squats, lunges, and sit-ups, employ the individual's own body weight as resistance. Push-ups, squats, lunges, leg lifts, and planks are examples of bodyweight exercises.
2. **Classic strength training** implements such as dumbbells, barbells, and kettlebells are examples of free weights. Lunges, squats, bench presses, and bent-over rows are just a few of the workouts that may be done with free weights.

Basic Resistance Training Techniques

Resistance Bands: These are little, portable items that produce resistance when stretched. They occur in a variety of shapes and sizes, such as rubber bands or tubes, sometimes with handles and attachments, and occasionally as a continuous ring. Resistance bands can be used for bicep curls, tricep extensions, shoulder presses, and chest presses, among other activities.

Weight machines are stationary equipment with a predetermined level of resistance. Weight machines may be used for several workouts, including chest presses, leg presses, shoulder presses, and leg curls.

When beginning resistance training, it is critical to select the appropriate exercises and resistance to guarantee safety and efficacy. It is best to work with a fitness expert or a qualified trainer to create a specific resistance training program that is suited to your fitness objectives and skills. Furthermore, to avoid injury and optimize the advantages of resistance training, it is critical to warm up before exercising, employ good form and technique, and cool down afterward.

Examples of Resistance Training Exercises for Teen Boys

Resistance training is a wonderful approach for teen males to increase their strength, improve their athletic performance, and improve their general fitness. Here are some examples of resistance training activities appropriate for adolescent boys:

- **Squats**: Squats are a lower-body complex exercise that works the quadriceps, hamstrings, and glutes. They may be done with your own bodyweight, free weights, or weight machines.

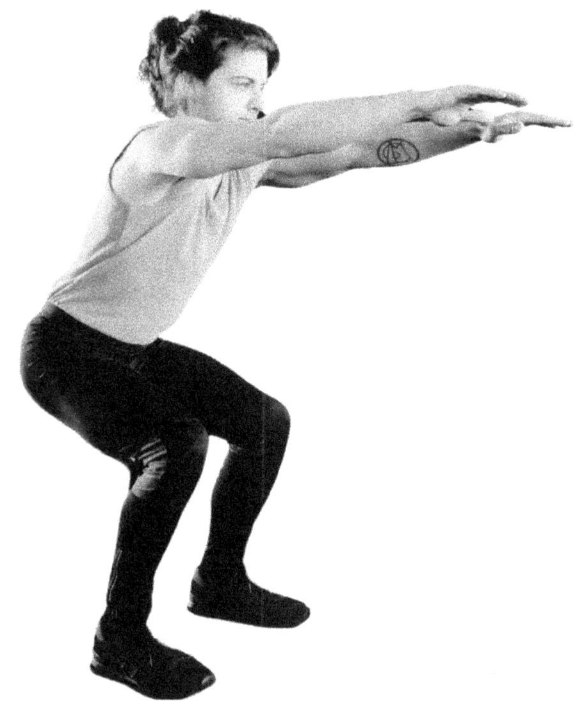

How To:
1. Stand upright with your feet hip-width apart at the beginning.
2. Engage your core by tightening your stomach muscles.

Squatting: To maintain balance, shift your weight over your heels.

3. At the same time, bend your knees and tilt forward at the hips.
4. Push your hips back and lower yourself as if sitting in an unseen chair.
5. Make sure your back, neck, and head are all in a neutral posture.
6. Keep your knees from folding in and from dropping over your toes.
7. To get back to standing, engage your glutes and core while pushing through your heels.
8. At the height of the action, fully extend your knees.

Maintaining good form and avoiding typical faults such as allowing the knees to sink in, not leading with the hips, and not engaging the core are critical.

Additionally, concentrating on glute activation and utilizing variants such as squat therapy might aid in the improvement of your squatting technique.

- **Bench Press:** A traditional workout that works the chest, shoulders, and triceps. It is possible to do it using a barbell, dumbbells, or weight machines.
  How To:
    1. Lie back on a level seat with your feet firmly planted on the ground.
    2. Pull your shoulder blades back and grab the bar with a narrow, overhand grip to limit the weight's line of travel.

Lowering the Bar:

1. Breathe in and slowly lower the bar until it reaches the center of your chest.

2. Keep your elbows tucked in and focus on working your chest muscles.
3. Driving your feet into the floor to engage your quadriceps and glutes when pressing the bar
4. Return the bar to the beginning position while concentrating on stimulating your chest, delts, and triceps.
5. As you press the bar up, exhale firmly.

Maintaining appropriate form and avoiding typical faults like arching your back too much, flaring your elbows out, and not keeping your feet firmly on the ground are critical.

Furthermore, utilizing a spotter or safety bars can assist avoid damage while still allowing you to push yourself to your limits

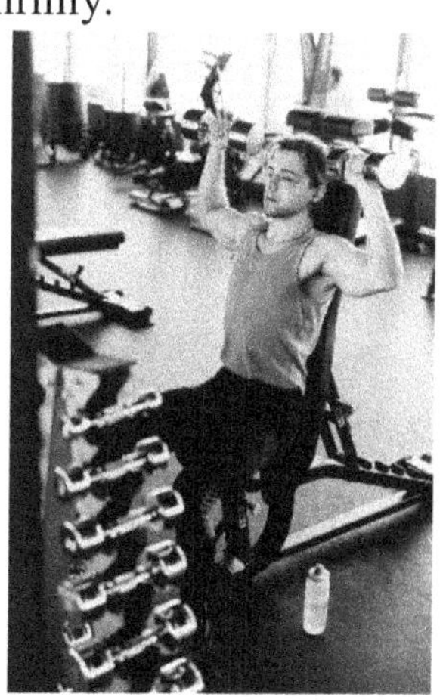

- **Deadlifts** are a complex exercise that focuses on the lower back, glutes, and hamstrings. They can be done with a barbell or dumbbells.

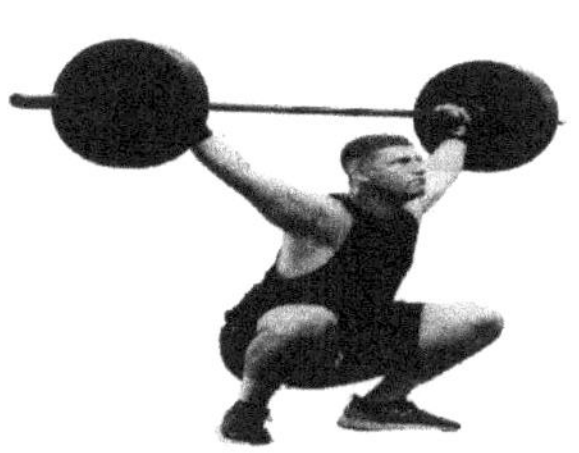

How To:

1. Place your feet shoulder-width apart behind a barbell.
2. Sit back with your hips, gently bend your knees, and lean forward with a firm core and flat back. Place your hands

shoulder-width apart on the bar, palms facing in toward your body.

3. Stand tall by pressing your feet into the floor and dragging your weight with you while maintaining your arms straight. At the peak, bring your hips forward and compress your core and glutes.
4. Return the weight to the floor by slowly reversing the movement, bending your knees and pushing your buttocks back. Maintain a flat back and keep the bar close to your body the entire time.

- Military Press: The military press is a shoulder and triceps-targeting workout. It is possible to do it using a barbell, dumbbells, or resistance bands.

How To:
1. Standing with your feet shoulder-width apart, hold the bar in an overhand grip that is slightly broader than shoulder-width.
2. Keep your elbows in front of the bar and your upper arms parallel to the ground as you lift the bar to your collarbone.

Pressing the Bar:

1. Maintain a neutral spine by bracing your core.
2. Extend your arms and press the bar overhead, ensuring that the movement originates from the shoulders and arms and not the rest of your body.
3. At the height of the exercise, fully extend your arms without locking out your elbows.

Raising the Bar:

1. Slowly lower the bar back to its starting position while maintaining control and using your core.

It's critical to maintain appropriate form and avoid typical faults like lifting the weight with momentum, arching your back, or flaring your elbows out to the sides.

Furthermore, beginning with a little weight and focusing on steady growth might help you master the exercise safely and successfully.

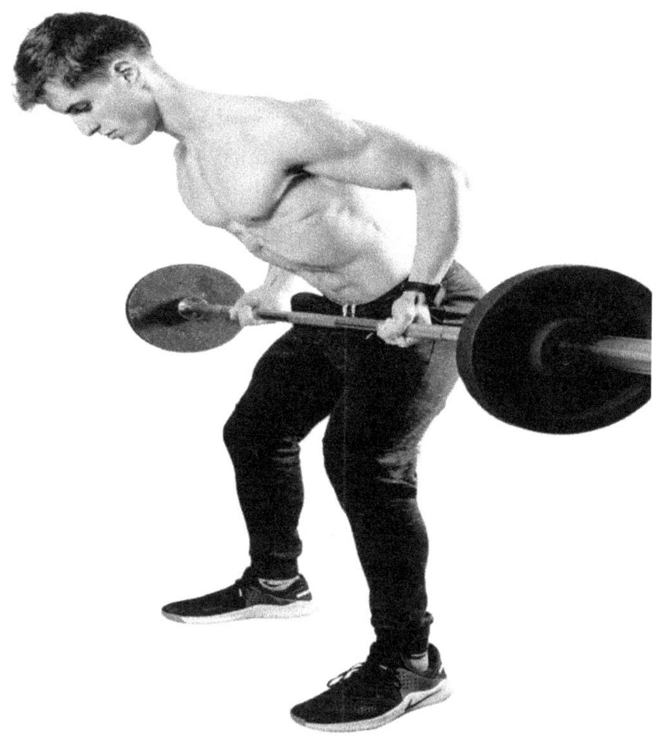

- **Pull-ups**: A bodyweight workout that works the back, biceps, and forearms. They may be done with a pull-up bar or with resistance bands.

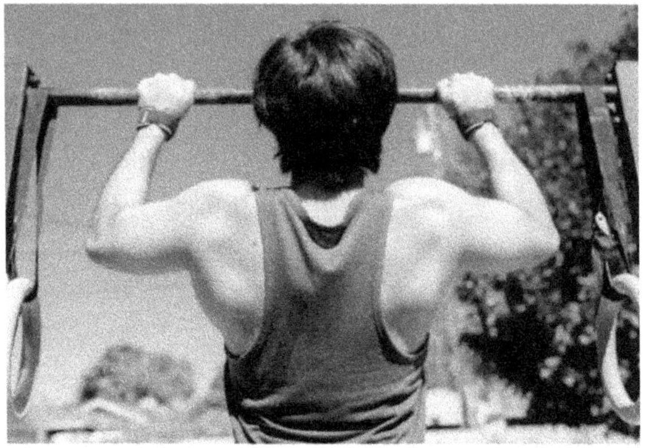

How To:

✓ Stand beneath a pull-up bar and hold it with an overhand grip that is slightly broader than shoulder width.
✓ Hang from the bar, arms fully extended and feet off the ground.

Taking a Step Up:

✓ Pull your body up towards the bar by using your back muscles and maintaining your elbows close to your body.
✓ Pull with your back muscles, not just your arms.
✓ Throughout the action, keep your core engaged and your body straight.

Bringing It Down:
✓ Slowly lower your body back to the starting position while maintaining control and engaging your core.

✓ Maintaining perfect form and avoiding typical faults like as swinging your body, not completely extending your arms at the bottom of the exercise, or not lifting your chin over the bar are all key.

Furthermore, beginning with the proper grip and focusing on steady progression will help you master the exercise safely and successfully.

- **Push-ups** are a bodyweight exercise that focuses on the chest, shoulders, and triceps. They may be done anywhere and can be tailored to specific fitness levels.

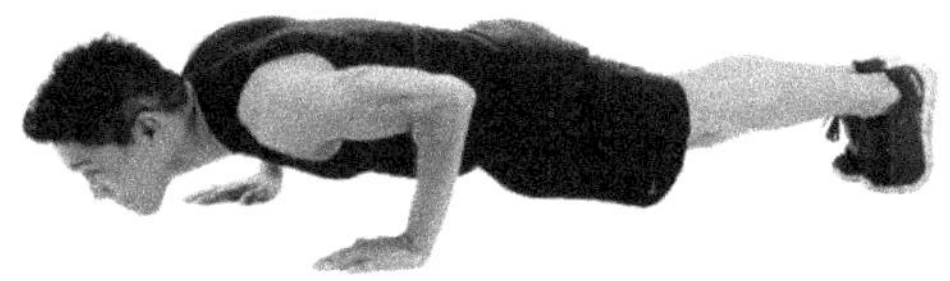

- **Lunges:** Lunges are a lower-body complex exercise that targets the quadriceps, hamstrings, and glutes. They may be done with your own bodyweight, free weights, or resistance bands.

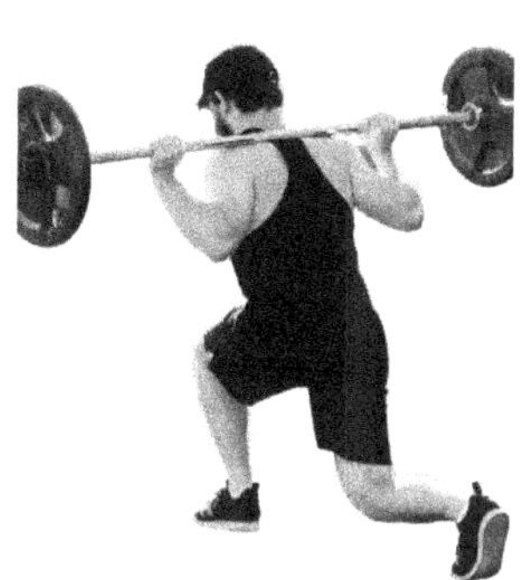

These examples illustrate the adaptability of resistance training activities appropriate for adolescent males. To guarantee successful and safe training, pick routines that correlate with individual fitness goals and abilities, and stress good form and technique.

Proper Warm-up and Cool-down Routines

Warm-up and cool-down procedures are critical for teen males participating in weight training activities. Here are some pointers for good warm-up and cool-down routines:

Warm-up: Before beginning any resistance training activity, perform a warm-up. Light aerobic activity, such as running or jumping jacks, should be used to boost heart rate and blood supply to the muscles.

Dynamic stretching, which involves moving the joints through their complete range of motion to prepare the muscles for activity, can also be included in a warm-up.

After finishing resistance training activities, a cool-down should be performed. Light aerobic activity, such as walking or cycling, should be used to progressively reduce heart rate and blood supply to the muscles.

Static stretching, which involves holding a stretch for 10-30 seconds to enhance flexibility and minimize muscular pain, can also be used in a cool-down.

Gradual Progression: As the strength of the resistance training exercises increases, gradually increase the intensity of the warm-up and cool-down routines.

Correct Form and Technique: To minimize injury and maximize the benefits of resistance training, use good form and technique throughout warm-up and cool-down exercises.

Hydration: To keep hydrated, drink lots of water before, during, and after weight training sessions.

Rest and Recovery: Allow time between resistance training sessions for rest and recovery to avoid injury and encourage muscular growth.

Teen males may ensure they have an efficient warm-up and cool-down regimen that complements their weight training workouts by following these guidelines. Proper warm-up and cool-down practices can aid in injury prevention, performance enhancement, and general health and well-being.

"Strength training is the canvas; you are the artist. Brush by brush, rep by rep, create a masterpiece. Build a foundation so unshakable that even your doubts will bow to your resilience."

CHAPTER 4

Safety First: Guidelines and Precautions

Teen males should emphasize safety when engaging in resistance training activities to reduce the chance of injury and provide a pleasurable experience. Here are some suggestions and safeguards to keep in mind:

✓ Examine the following items: Check any equipment for damage or wear and tear before utilizing it. Check that it is in good working order and that it has been properly maintained.

✓ Examine the Location: Examine the location where you will be exercising for potential risks such as uneven surfaces or barriers.

✓ Understand Emergency Numbers: Understand how to call emergency numbers in the event of an accident or injury.

✓ Follow the following safety procedures: Understand the company's safety policies and procedures, as well as the HSE golden guidelines.

✓ Wear suitable Clothing and Shoes: To avoid injury, wear suitable clothing and shoes for the workout.

✓ Use good Form and Technique: To minimize injury and maximize the benefits of resistance training, use good form and technique throughout exercises.

✓ Begin slowly by using lesser weights and fewer repetitions, gradually increasing intensity as you gain strength and familiarity with the movements.

✓ Stay Hydrated: To stay hydrated, drink lots of water before, during, and after weight training sessions.

✓ Warm-up and cool-down: To avoid injury and optimize the benefits of resistance training, warm up before beginning any strength training activity and cool down afterward.

✓ Pay Attention to Your Body: Pay heed to your body's cues and avoid overdoing it, which might raise your chance of injury.

Understanding Your Body's Limits

Knowing your body's limits is essential before engaging in any physical activity, including resistance training. It entails recognizing the limits of physical and mental exertion in order to avoid harm and improve general well-being. Below are some critical insights about your body's limits:

- Body Sufficiency: Because the body has temporal boundaries, it is a susceptible and decomposable entity. It is critical to recognize that the body has limits, and adhering to these limits is critical for long-term health and injury avoidance.

- Considerations Regarding Age: As people become older, their bodies change, which might affect their physical performance and recuperation. Recognizing and reacting to these changes is critical for personalizing training programs to the body's ever-changing constraints.

- Mind-Body Connection: The mind is important in establishing the boundaries of the body. According to research, the brain determines endurance and pain tolerance, emphasizing the interrelated nature of mental and physical constraints.

- Paying Attention to Body cues: Understanding the body's limits requires paying attention to cues such as weariness, discomfort, and pain. Ignoring these indications can result in overexertion and damage, thus it is critical to respect and listen to the body's messages.

- Pushing Boundaries Safely: Recognizing limitations is crucial, but safely pushing boundaries via progressive development and adaptability may lead to physical and mental growth. This should be done mindfully and with an appreciation of one's own capabilities.

Common Injuries and Prevention Strategies

Sprains, strains, joint injuries (such as knee, shoulder, and ankle injuries), muscle injuries, dislocations, fractures, Achilles tendon injuries, and soreness along the shin bone are all common sports injuries among teen males participating in resistance training or other physical activity. It is critical to follow safety rules and best practices in order to avoid severe injuries. Some significant injury prevention measures include:

- **Proper warm-up and cool-down**: Proper warm-up and cool-down practices before and after exercise can help prepare the body for physical activity and lower the chance of injury.
- **Strength Training and Flexibility**: Incorporating strength training and flexibility activities into a fitness regimen will help reduce the likelihood of injury.
- **Hydration is vital for maintaining health and reducing cramping.** It is critical to keep hydrated before, during, and after exercise.
- **Wearing the Right Gear**: Wearing suitable and well fitting protective equipment, such as pads, helmets, mouthguards, and eyeglasses, can assist prevent injuries during physical exercise

- **Good Technique:** Using good technique during exercise and sports activities can help lessen the chance of injury.
- **Rest and recovery:** Taking at least one day off per week and at least one month off per year from training enables the body to recuperate and can help prevent overuse issues.
- Teen males can lower their risk of common sports injuries and stay safe and healthy while participating in physical exercise and resistance training by following these injury prevention measures.

Importance of Supervision and Form

It is impossible to overestimate the significance of monitoring and form in resistance training. Supervision offers direction, assistance, and responsibility to ensure that activities are done appropriately and safely. It also aids in injury prevention and maximization of training effects. Correct form is critical for targeting the proper muscles and avoiding strain or damage. Here are a few highlight:

In an Organizational Context, Supervision: Supervision in an organizational environment entails training, leading, monitoring, and observing personnel while they execute their duties. It is critical for sustaining group cohesiveness, communicating instructions, and facilitating control.

Managerial Supervision: In a managerial environment, supervision include addressing workload, encouraging worker well-being, and fostering staff growth. It holds both the management and the employee accountable and is essential for motivating and mentoring employees to accomplish organizational goals.

The Importance of Supervision: The importance of supervision lies in ensuring that subordinates are functioning efficiently and successfully. It serves as a critical link between workers and management by offering employee training and keeping interpersonal interaction with workers.

Benefits of Effective Supervision: There are several advantages to effective supervision for both the supervisee and the supervisor. It can aid in the development of professional relationships as well as the establishment of an organizational culture of honesty, critical assessment, and learning. It also promotes contemplation, aids in job advancement, and boosts confidence and critical thinking.

Monitoring and perfect form are critical in resistance training to guarantee that exercises are executed correctly, to avoid injuries, and to optimize the advantages of the training. Whether in an organizational or management setting, supervision is critical in directing, encouraging, and inspiring employees to achieve their objectives.

"In the realm of strength, foundations matter. Lay yours with passion, commitment, and the clang of weights. The stronger your base, the higher your ascent. Rise, teenage titans!"

CHAPTER 5

Strength Training for Sports and Fitness

Strength training for sports and fitness is necessary for adolescent males because it improves athletic performance, builds strength, and improves endurance, speed, and overall sporting performance.

Here are a few highlights

Strength Training Benefits for Teen Boys: Strength training prevents overtraining, increases exercise economy, improves aerobic endurance performance, and aids in the development of dynamic athletic performance.

Goblet squats, barbell squats, barbell bench press, bent-over barbell row, military press, and stiff-leg deadlifts are some excellent strength-training exercises for teen boys.

Fitness Plan for teens: Exercises like as bench press, hip thrust, Romanian deadlift, chin-ups, and others might be included in an example fitness plan for teens.

Considerations for Pre- and Post-Adolescent Boys: Strength training should differ for teens who have not yet reached puberty and those who have. Bodyweight training and other movement-based workouts should be prioritized for pre-pubertal teens, while a resistance training program should be undertaken for post-pubertal teenagers.

Training Frequency and Duration: Teenagers should ideally train three days a week, using full-body workouts, to allow for adequate recovery and growth.

Teen males may increase their sports performance, grow lean muscle, and improve their overall athletic ability by including strength training into their fitness program. To guarantee successful and safe strength training, pick exercises that correlate with individual fitness goals and abilities, and emphasis good form and technique.

Tailoring Workouts for Specific Sports

Tailoring exercises for certain sports for teen boys entails creating a strength training program that is tailored to their specific demands, goals, and circumstances, taking their sport and position into account.

Here are a few highlights:

- Strength Training for Specific Sports: Sport-specific strength training regimens are designed to meet the unique requirements of each sport. These programs are designed to improve the athlete's capacity to apply force in their sport while also ensuring that the strength training exercises are as close to the real sports movements as feasible.
- Strength training aids in the prevention of overtraining, increases exercise economy, improves aerobic endurance performance, and aids in the development of dynamic athletic performance.
- Goblet squats, barbell squats, barbell bench press, bent-over barbell row, military press, and stiff-leg deadlifts are examples of excellent strength training exercises.
- Fitness Plan for teens: Exercises like as bench press, hip thrust, Romanian deadlift, chin-ups, and others might be included in an example fitness plan for teens.

- Training Frequency and Duration: Teenagers should ideally train three days a week, using full-body workouts, to allow for adequate recovery and growth.

Cross-Training Benefits

Cross-training has various advantages for adolescent guys, including:

- Prevention and Rehabilitation of Injuries: Cross-training can aid in injury prevention and recovery by encouraging athletes to employ a variety of muscle groups and movement patterns, hence lowering the chance of overuse injuries.
- Improved Cardiovascular Endurance: Cross-training can improve cardiovascular endurance, which is important for general health and fitness.
- Cross-training helps players to target muscle areas that are not used in their major sport, resulting in a more well-rounded and adaptable athlete.
- Cross-training may give much-needed healing time from the major activity while also keeping players cognitively engaged during their off-season or when taking a vacation from their main sport.
- Cross-training allows players to learn new abilities and adapt to other sports, which can help with overall athletic growth and skill acquisition.
- Weight Management: Cross-training exercises can help teen males maintain a healthy weight by burning calories and working off surplus energy.
- Cross-training can assist athletes stay in shape and ready to return to their major sport when the season begins by helping them maintain fitness levels throughout the off-season.

Balancing Strength and Cardiovascular Fitness

The ability to balance strength and cardiovascular fitness is critical for general health and sports success. Here are some significant takeaways

- Injury Avoidance: By enhancing muscle strength, endurance, and general physical conditioning, balancing strength and cardiovascular fitness can help prevent injuries.
- Improved Endurance and Strength: Cardio exercises like jogging and cycling increase endurance, while strength exercises like weightlifting increase strength and balance. Both forms of exercise, when combined, can assist avoid injury and enhance general fitness.
- planned sessions: Progress in both aerobic and strength training is feasible if sessions are planned and tailored to balance both forms of exercise.
- The importance of balance: The balance of aerobic and strength training is determined by individual goals. Someone seeking to bodybuilding, for example, will have a different workout schedule than someone looking to reduce weight. The necessity of balancing the two workouts is determined by the workout aim.
- Sport-Specific Training: Strength training is an integral component of fitness for almost every athlete. Strength training has numerous and huge benefits for sports performance. It is not simply an essential conditioning component for power sportsmen like football and rugby.

It is critical to balance strength and cardiovascular fitness for injury prevention, enhanced endurance and strength, and overall sports performance. The appropriate balance is determined by individual goals as well as the unique demands of the sport or activity.

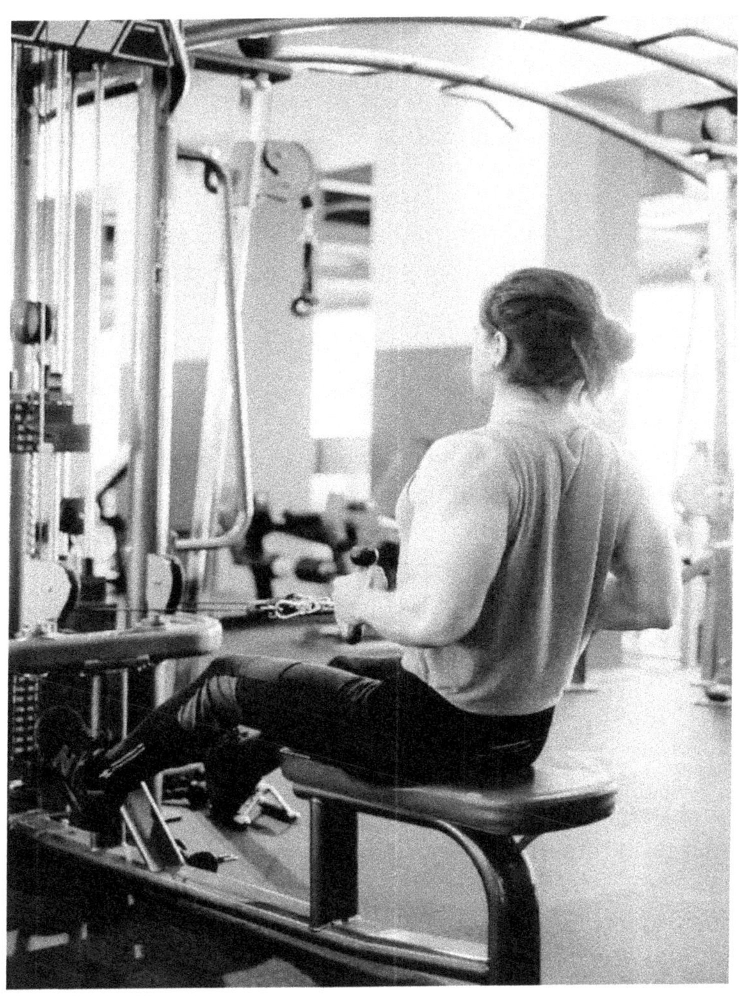

CHAPTER 6

Mind and Body Connection

Incorporating mind-body activities into a teen boy's training program can provide several benefits to his physical and mental health. Here are some advantages of adding mind-body exercises into an adolescent boy's training routine:

- Stress and Anxiety Reduction: Yoga and other mind-body activities help reduce anxiety and enhance mental health in both healthy youth and those with mental health difficulties.
- Improved Mental Health: Regular exercise has been shown to lower stress and anxiety, as well as boost brain health and learning.
- Physical Health Improvement: Exercise improves every area of the body, including the mind. It can help people maintain a healthy weight, lessen their risk of certain illnesses, and strengthen their bones.
- Improved Athletic Performance: Mind-body activities may improve speed and response time, as well as teach balance and provide a cognitive challenge.
- Mind-body workouts allow players to learn new skills and adapt to diverse sports, which can benefit overall athletic growth and skill acquisition.

Incorporating mind-body activities into a teen boy's training program can help him develop better body awareness, increase emotional management, and improve his overall athletic performance. Encouragement of a combination of strength training, cardiovascular fitness, and mind-body activities can assist teen males in maintaining a healthy lifestyle and attaining optimal physical and mental well-being.

Mental Resilience and Confidence

Mental resilience and confidence are critical for adolescent males' general well-being and performance in a variety of areas, including academics, athletics, and personal relationships. Here are some significant takeaways

- Confidence and self-belief: A strong trust in oneself is at the basis of resilience, and confidence is a fundamental attribute. Teen guys who are self-assured and confident are more likely to recover from setbacks and challenges.
- Solid Objectives and Commitment: Another important quality of resilient people is the ability to set and achieve goals. Teen guys who develop and commit to objectives are more likely to succeed and gain confidence.
- Improved Mental Health: Positive psychology qualities such as resilience and self-esteem are essential indications of positive mental health. Individuals with resilience can cope with adversity and stress, whereas self-esteem encourages self-acceptance, self-responsibility, and self-maintenance.
- Social Support: Another crucial aspect in developing resilience and self-esteem is social support. Teen boys who have positive, supportive interactions and networks are more likely to develop resilience and confidence.
- Building Resilience: Being able to adjust to life's tragedies and setbacks is part of building resilience. Teen males may develop resilience by setting objectives, cultivating a positive mentality, finding social support, and engaging in self-care activities.

Stress Management through Exercise

Exercise is an excellent stress-reduction strategy for adolescent guys. Regular physical exercise helps lower stress hormones and increase endorphin synthesis, which aids in relaxing.

Here are some of the primary advantages of including exercise into a stress management program for adolescent boys:

- Stress and Anxiety Reduction: Exercise can lower stress and anxiety in adolescent males by giving a break from stressors and enhancing the body's response to stress.
- Exercise can benefit teen males' mental health by lowering depression, enhancing cognitive performance, and fostering relaxation.
- Physical Health Improvement: Exercise improves every area of the body, including the mind. It can assist teen males in maintaining a healthy weight, lowering their risk of certain illnesses, and improving bone strength.
- Improved Athletic Performance: Exercise can improve teen males' athletic performance by increasing endurance, strength, and balance.
- Versatility and adaptability: Physical activity allows adolescent males to learn new skills and adapt to new sports, which can be advantageous for overall athletic development and skill acquisition.
- Exercise can help teen males acquire better stress management skills, improve their mental and physical health, and increase their overall sports performance when included in a stress management program. Encouragement of a combination of strength training, cardiovascular fitness, and mind-body activities can

assist teen males in maintaining a healthy lifestyle and attaining optimal physical and mental well-being.

The Role of Strength Training in Mental Well-being

Strength training is important for enhancing mental health, especially in adolescent guys. Various investigations and research have revealed the following advantages:

✓ Strength training has been demonstrated to boost self-esteem in healthy younger and older persons, as well as in people undergoing cardiac rehabilitation and those suffering from depression.
✓ Stress and Anxiety Reduction: Strength training can reduce stress and anxiety by reducing levels of the stress hormone cortisol.
✓ Resistance exercise, such as strength training, has been demonstrated in studies to improve cognition, self-esteem, and depression, hence contributing to anxiolytic effects.
✓ Strength training is regarded as a natural antidepressant, with research showing that it can help prevent and treat depression.
✓ Strength training has been related to increased sleep quality, cognitive function, and tiredness reduction, all of which contribute to overall mental well-being.

CHAPTER 7

Lifestyle Integration and Future Growth

Teen male strength training requires lifestyle integration as well as future growth considerations. Strength training is usually regarded as beneficial to children's and teens' health, fitness, and athletic performance. Youth, or the interval between childhood and adulthood, is an important time for strength training and is often considered optimal for young athletes. Strength training tends to develop muscle strength, power, and endurance in children and adolescents, with teenage gains outperforming preadolescent gains.

Strength training has also been demonstrated in studies to enhance quantitative health markers in children, including cardiovascular fitness, body composition, blood lipid profiles, and insulin sensitivity.

When it comes to future growth, incorporating resistance training into kid fitness programs is crucial. When done correctly, strength training may be beneficial to teens and even pre-adolescents. However, supervision by a certified expert is required, and a fitness evaluation and a safe program suited to individual needs and goals are recommended. To ensure the safety and usefulness of the training, it is also necessary to choose a structured, well-supervised program or a qualified teacher.

When it comes to lifestyle integration, it is crucial to give age-appropriate workouts, build ideal movement patterns, and target important muscle groups. Teen boys should consider their goals and what they hope to gain from strength training. Furthermore, it is recommended to avoid supplements and instead focus on a well-rounded program that incorporates activities such as bicycling, running, and flexibility exercises in addition to strength training.

Creating Sustainable Habits

Developing long-term habits in boys' strength training is critical for long-term success. To develop long-term fitness habits, it is necessary to gradually incorporate them into daily life, adding a new habit once every week or two weeks.

For example, if a guy is new to exercise, he may focus on developing a regular walking habit and setting weekly goals for distance and number of steps, progressively boosting stamina.

To guarantee the safety and efficacy of strength training, it is important to locate an organized, well-supervised program or a trained teacher.

Individual requirements and goals should be addressed, and age-appropriate exercises should be provided, teaching good movement patterns and treating important muscle groups.

To develop long-term habits, it is critical to focus on long-term objectives and total well-being, avoiding supplements and focusing on a well-rounded program that includes not just strength training but other activities such as bicycling, jogging, and flexibility exercises.

Consistency is essential for developing long-term habits in boys' strength training. It is critical to consider training like an essential errand and to prioritize consistency over intensity.

Rest is also important for growth, and taking enough of it can help you get most out of your workouts.

Tracking and Celebrating Progress

Tracking and rewarding improvement is a vital part of boys' strength training. Tracking progress may be a great source of motivation since it allows people to track their success and adapt their strategies accordingly.

There are a variety of practical and imaginative techniques for measuring progress, such as logging training sessions, taking periodic images of the physique, and charting repetitions and weights in each exercise.

It is critical to celebrate each milestone, whether it is gaining strength, endurance, flexibility, or general well-being, in order to develop lasting habits.

Setting up a reward system for attaining milestones may also be a powerful motivation.

Keeping a journal, taking photographs, or using a fitness app to track progress can also help people remember how far they've come.

Sharing fitness objectives with a friend, family member, or gym companion who can serve as an accountability partner may also be a powerful motivation.

Resources for Continued Learning and Growth

There are several options accessible to guys for continuous learning and progress in strength training. The National

Strength and Conditioning Association (NSCA) is one organization that provides evidence-based tools and resources for strength and conditioning practitioners.

The National Federation of High Schools Learning Center also provides a Strength and Conditioning Course through the NSCA.

Another useful resource is the American Council on Exercise (ACE), which provides a strength training handbook for parents and instructors.

The study discusses the advantages of strength training for children as well as advice for safe and successful training.

Bodybuilding.com also provides men with sustainable fitness ideas, such as advice on developing sustainable training routines.

The website highlights the significance of approaching training like a necessary errand, prioritizing consistency over intensity, and receiving adequate rest.

Horizon provides a blog article about how to stay motivated and master fitness objectives for long-term success.

The post offers advice on how to create S.M.A.R.T. goals, measure progress, and sustain motivation through various training and reward systems.

Tips for Staying Motivated To Continue Strength Training

Long-term success requires being motivated to maintain strength training. Based on the search results, here are some suggestions:

- ❖ Practice positive self-talk: Remind yourself of your achievements and the advantages of strength exercise.
- ❖ Discover a new motivation to work out: Concentrate on the benefits of strength training, such as increased health or personal success.
- ❖ Change things up: Include variation in your workouts to keep them interesting and fun.
- ❖ Find a workout partner who is more fit than you: Training alongside someone more experienced might inspire you to strive harder.
- ❖ Set specific and attainable goals: To measure your progress and stay motivated, set S.M.A.R.T. goals (Specific, Measurable, Assignable, Realistic, Time-Based).
- ❖ Prioritize consistency over intensity: Rather than pushing yourself too hard, too fast, focus on establishing a steady routine.
- ❖ Include physical activity in your daily routine: Schedule your workouts on particular days of the week to establish a habit.
- ❖ Join a group or a class: Take part in social activities or exercise courses to keep yourself motivated and accountable.
- ❖ Reward yourself: For hitting milestones, treat yourself to a cheat meal or new training gear.
- ❖ Take a holistic approach to health: In order to enhance your strength training efforts, include appropriate eating and sleeping habits.

CONCLUSION

You've crossed the finish line, but the true trip has only just begun. You've discovered the keys to becoming a stronger, healthier, and more confident version of yourself. It is now time to put information into practice.

Don't let this book sit on a shelf collecting dust. Grab your workout bag, lace on your sneakers, and enter your prospective arena. Every rep, set, every drop of sweat is a testimonial to your dedication, a stone built in the foundation of your future self. Remember, Rome was not constructed in a day, and neither is the body of a Titan. However, each step taken, each hurdle overcome, puts you closer to your ultimate goal.

This book serves as your guide, coach, and cheerleader at the gym. But the true power is in your hands. So, what are you holding out for? Claim your power, your confidence, and your future. Buy "Strength Training for Teen Boys" today and discover your inner Titan!

And when you've achieved new heights, when you've broken through barriers, tell your tale. Leave an honest review of this book to assist other aspiring Titans in their initial steps toward greatness. Let us work together to create a legion of strong, confident boys who redefine what it means to be a man.

Buy now, conquer later, and remember that the only restriction you put for yourself is the one you make for yourself.

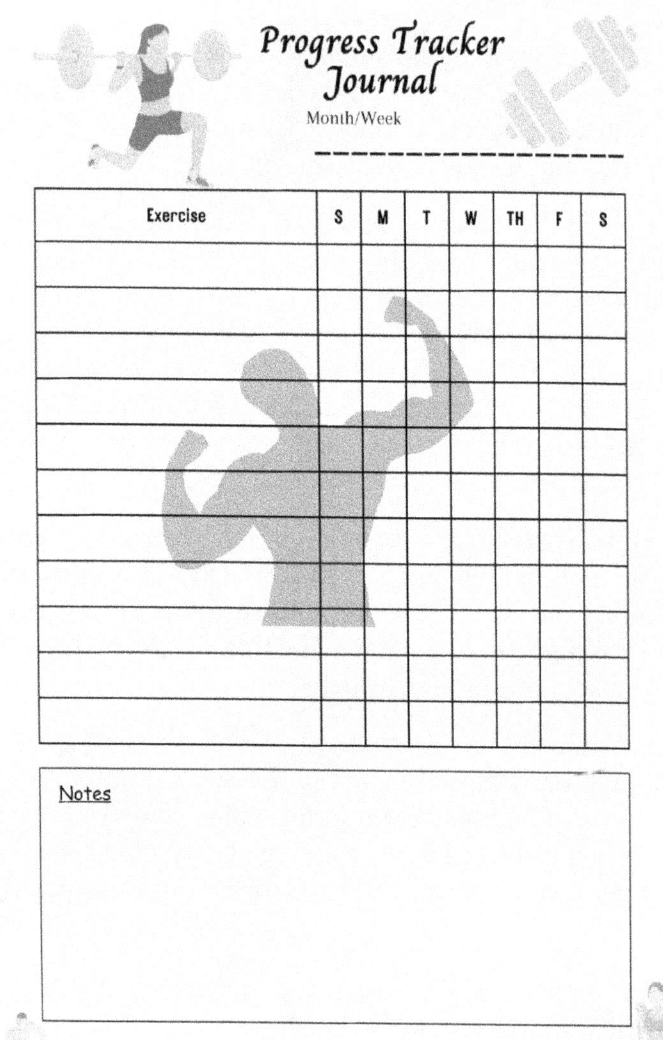

Exercise	S	M	T	W	TH	F	S

Notes

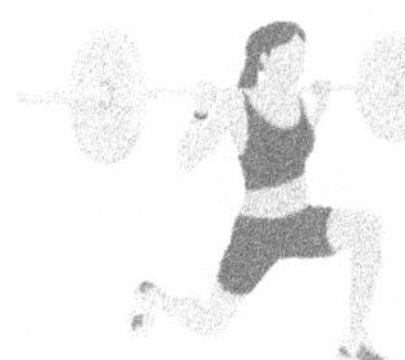

Progress Tracker Journal

Month/Week

____

Exercise	S	M	T	W	TH	F	S

Notes

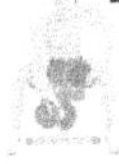
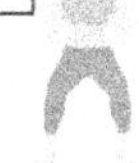

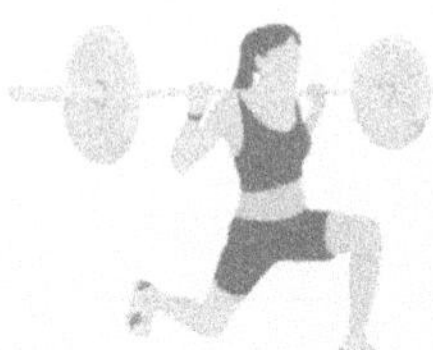

Progress Tracker
Journal

Month/Week
____

Exercise	S	M	T	W	TH	F	S

<u>Notes</u>

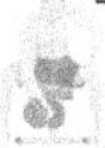
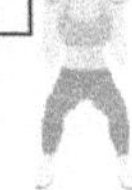

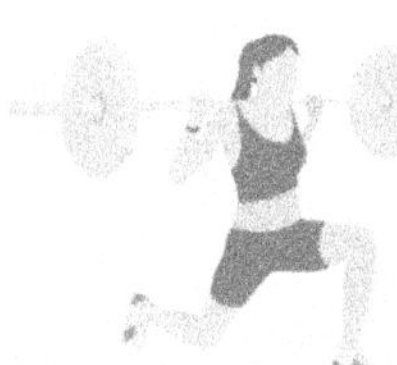

Progress Tracker
Journal

Month/Week

____

Exercise	S	M	T	W	TH	F	S

Notes

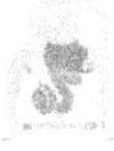
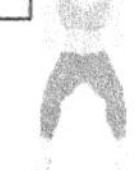

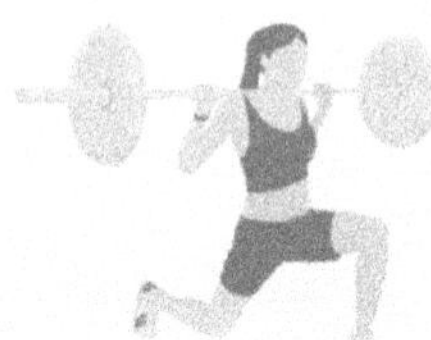

Progress Tracker Journal

Month/Week

____

Exercise	S	M	T	W	TH	F	S

<u>Notes</u>

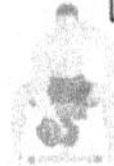
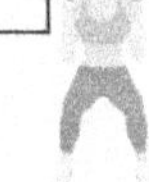

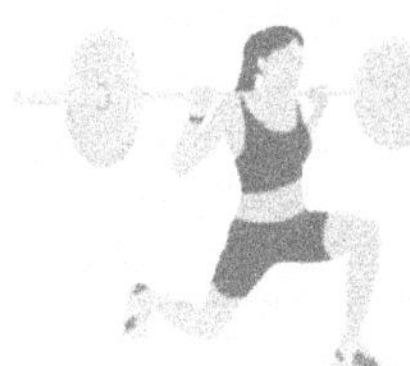

Progress Tracker
Journal

Month/Week

____

Exercise	S	M	T	W	TH	F	S

Notes

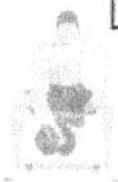
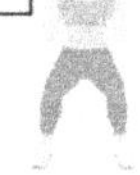

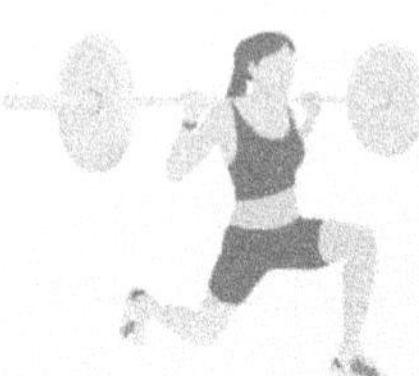

Progress Tracker
Journal

Month/Week

____

Exercise	S	M	T	W	TH	F	S

<u>Notes</u>

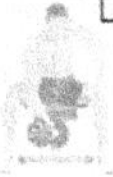

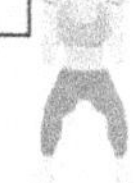

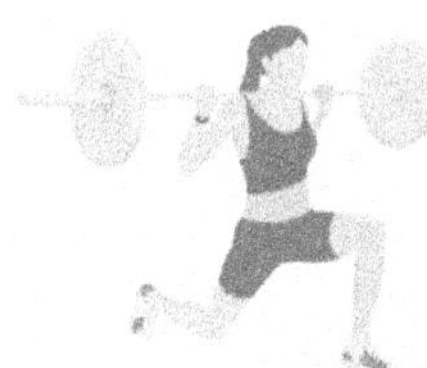

Progress Tracker
Journal

Month/Week

____

Exercise	S	M	T	W	TH	F	S

<u>Notes</u>

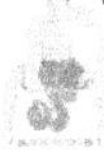
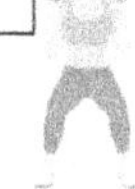

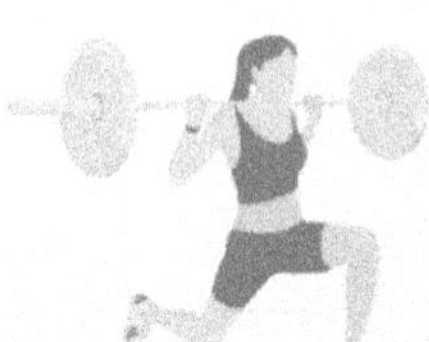

Progress Tracker
Journal

Month/Week

____

Exercise	S	M	T	W	TH	F	S

<u>Notes</u>

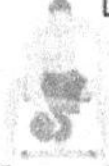
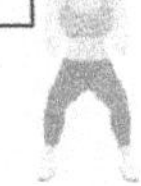

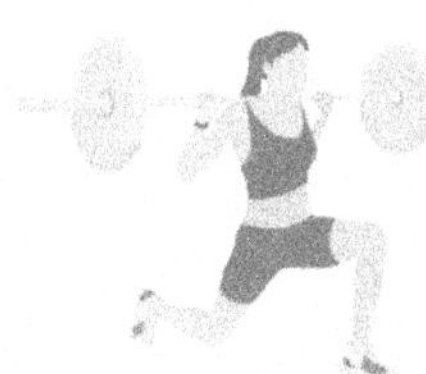

Progress Tracker Journal

Month/Week

____

Exercise	S	M	T	W	TH	F	S

<u>Notes</u>

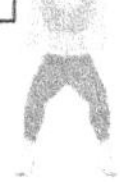

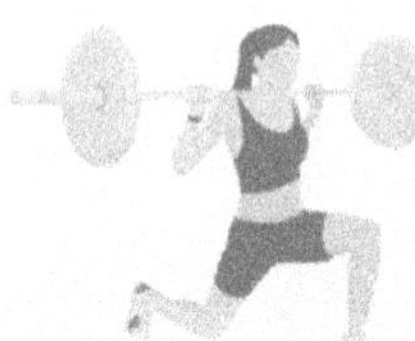

Progress Tracker
Journal

Month/Week

____

Exercise	S	M	T	W	TH	F	S

Notes

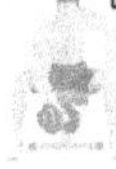
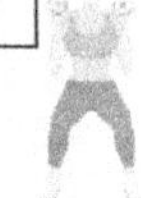

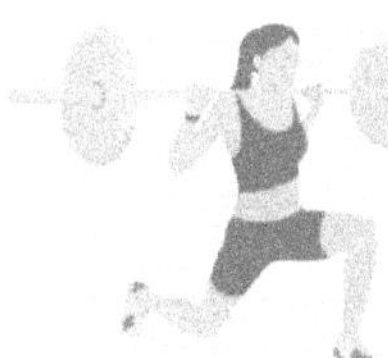

Progress Tracker Journal

Month/Week

____

Exercise	S	M	T	W	TH	F	S

Notes

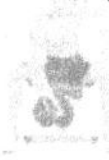
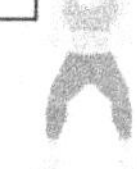

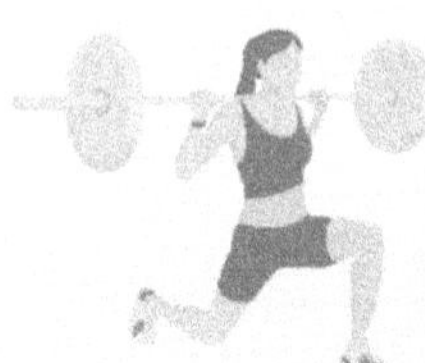

Progress Tracker
Journal

Month/Week

____

Exercise	S	M	T	W	TH	F	S

<u>Notes</u>

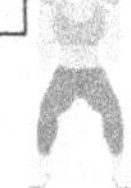

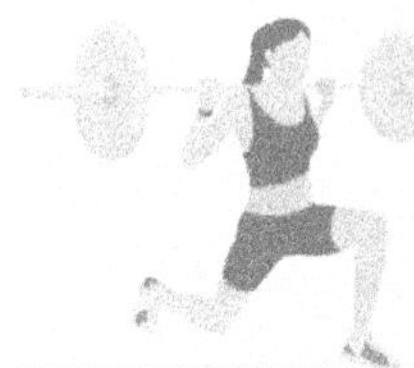

Progress Tracker
Journal

Month/Week

____

Exercise	S	M	T	W	TH	F	S

Notes

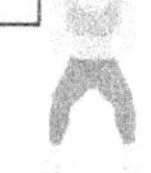

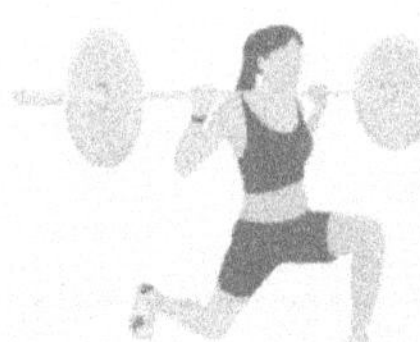

Progress Tracker
Journal

Month/Week

____

Exercise	S	M	T	W	TH	F	S

Notes

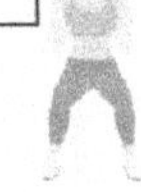

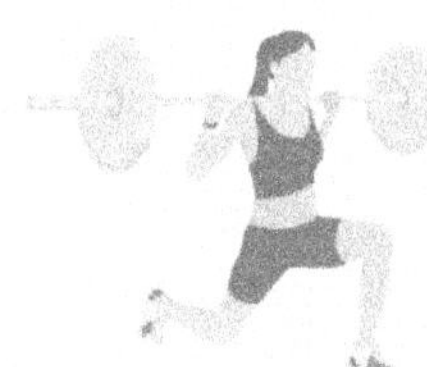

Progress Tracker
Journal

Month/Week

____

Exercise	S	M	T	W	TH	F	S

Notes

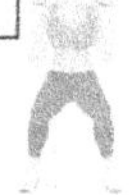

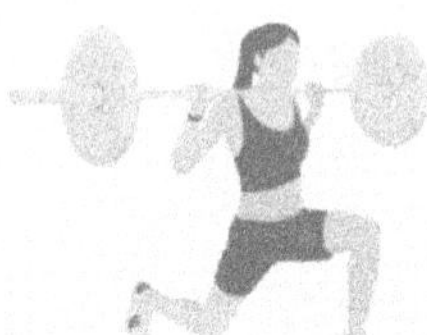

Progress Tracker
Journal

Month/Week
____

Exercise	S	M	T	W	TH	F	S

<u>Notes</u>

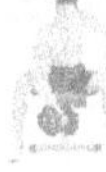
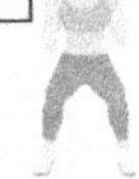

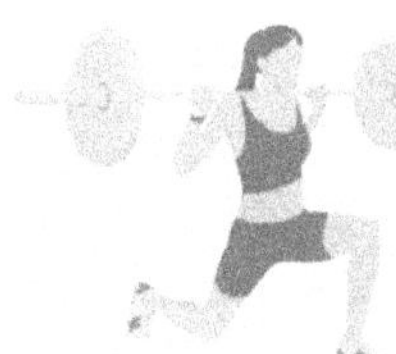

Progress Tracker
Journal

Month/Week

____

Exercise	S	M	T	W	TH	F	S

<u>Notes</u>

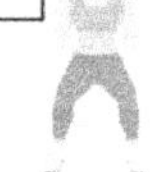

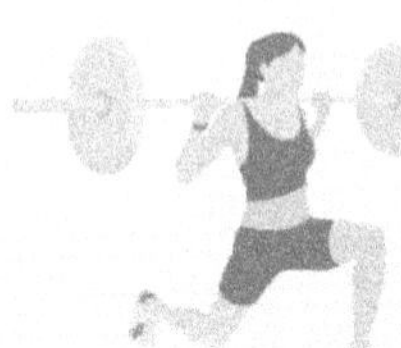

Progress Tracker
Journal

Month/Week

____

Exercise	S	M	T	W	TH	F	S

Notes

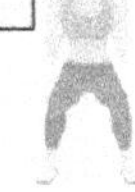

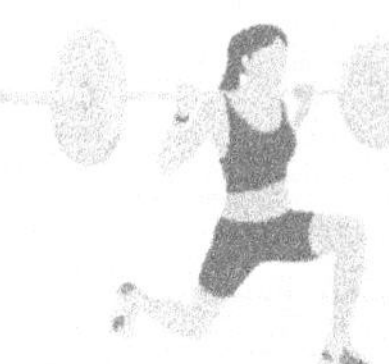

Progress Tracker
Journal

Month/Week

____

Exercise	S	M	T	W	TH	F	S

Notes

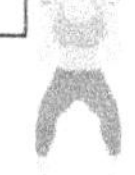

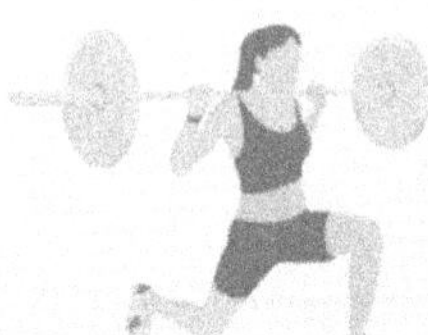

Progress Tracker
Journal

Month/Week

____

Exercise	S	M	T	W	TH	F	S

Notes

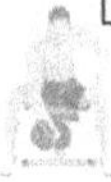
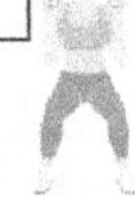